Skinnytaste Simple Cookbook

Quick and Wholesome Dishes with Minimal Ingredients.

By

Virgie W. Miller

Copyright

Introduction

We frequently find ourselves working against the clock while juggling work, family, and personal time in the hustle and bustle of modern life. The significance of keeping a balanced diet can easily be forgotten amid this frenzy. To save time, we turn to packaged snacks, takeout menus, and convenience foods. But what if I told you that you could enjoy wholesome, delicious meals without spending a lot of time in the kitchen? Hello and welcome to "Skinnytaste Simple Cookbook," your entryway to a world of healthy, quick meals that only require seven ingredients or less.

It's not necessary to be complicated to cook. It may even be delightfully straightforward. This cookbook is your ticket to the pleasure of cooking meals that are both healthy for your body and delicious. The recipes in these pages are created to make your culinary adventure simpler, more pleasurable, and more accessible than ever before, regardless of whether you're an experienced home cook or a kitchen newbie.

It's vital to take a step back and analyze the advantages of cooking at home in a society where we are constantly exposed to commercials for fast food and packaged convenience foods. The process of cooking a meal from scratch has an unmistakable allure, and the benefits go well beyond the dinner table.

Home-cooked meals typically tend to be healthier than their restaurant or packaged counterparts, according to research. You can choose the components that go into your meals when you cook at home. To satisfy your nutritional requirements, you can select fresh, high-quality ingredients and control portion proportions. An effective tool for controlling your health and well-being is this level of control.

Additionally, cooking at home may be a rewarding experience that helps you develop a closer relationship with the food you eat. You'll learn to relish the delight of a meal that is well-prepared and develop a deeper appreciation for the tastes and textures of various foods.

Despite the many benefits of cooking at home, it can be challenging to find the time and energy to prepare a healthy supper after a long day at work or a busy afternoon of errands. Naturally, it's not always easy. This is where "Skinnytaste Simple" can save the day.

The difficulties that many of us have when attempting to live a better lifestyle are addressed in this recipe. We recognize that you might not have the time to spend hours in the kitchen creating elaborate dishes or trawling upscale marketplaces for rare ingredients. We have chosen simplicity as our guiding concept because of this.

Like you, I had a hectic life and a desire to live a healthy lifestyle, which is how my adventure into the realm of straightforward, wholesome cuisine began. I encountered the same pressures and time restrictions that so many of us have every day as dedicated home cooks. Without compromising the priceless moments I could spend with my loved ones, I wanted to eat excellent meals.

This ambition sent me on a culinary quest in search of foods that were both nourishing and simple to make. I combed through cookbooks, tried several recipes, and eventually understood how wonderful meals could be made using only a few simple components. Along the way, I was motivated by the notion that cooking ought to be enjoyable and nourishing rather than a burdensome task.

Your experience through "Skinnytaste Simple Cookbook" will benefit from my years of research and experimentation. To ensure that each dish satisfies the standards of simplicity, wholesomeness, and, most importantly, deliciousness, it has been meticulously created. I put my entire being into creating these recipes, and I can't wait for you to discover the joy of simple cooking.

Are you prepared to accompany me into the kitchen now? Together, let's set out on this culinary journey where basic ingredients are transformed into mouth watering dishes and where eating healthily becomes more than just a choice but a wonderful way of life.

Kitchen requisites

Let's take time to study the fundamental components of your culinary journey before diving right into our collection of simple and healthy dishes. You, the home cook, will require a collection of tools and ingredients to produce your culinary masterpieces, much as a painter uses a palette of colors and brushes. Let's begin with the fundamentals.

Important Kitchen Tools

Imagine entering your kitchen like an experienced chef would, equipped with a toolbox that is ideal for the current culinary tasks. Even though you don't need a professional kitchen, a few essential items can greatly improve your ability to cook. The following kitchen necessities will make your experience with "Skinnytaste Simple Cookbook" even more enjoyable:

- **Sharp knives:** The foundation of any kitchen is a nice pair of sharp knives. Purchase a serrated knife, a paring knife, and a chef's knife. Sharpening them regularly promotes safe and effective cutting.

- **Cutting Boards:** Use bamboo, plastic, or wood cutting boards. They shield your surfaces while offering a firm surface for chopping, dicing, and slicing.

- **Dishes and pots:** It is imperative to have a solid collection of pots and pans in varied sizes. For simple cooking and cleanup, think about using nonstick skillets. For soups and stews, a heavy-bottomed pot is also a good idea.

- **Measuring Spoons and Cups** In cooking, exact measurements are essential. Have a set of measuring spoons and cups for smaller amounts of liquids and dry ingredients.

- **Mixing bowls:** For combining ingredients, marinating food, and preserving leftovers, having a selection of mixing bowls in various sizes is helpful.

- **Utensils:** For diverse cooking and stirring, equip your kitchen with spatulas, wooden spoons, tongs, and a ladle.

- **Baking pans and sheets:** Have baking sheets, cake pans, and muffin tins on hand if you enjoy baking.

- **Food processor or blender:**
  A blender or food processor
  can make chores like making
  smoothies, pureeing soups,
  or producing homemade
  sauces easier, however, they
  are not necessary.

- **Zester and the Grater:**
  These implements are ideal
  for garnishing your meals with
  freshly grated cheese and
  zest.

- **Strainer or colander:** Use this to strain sauces, drain pasta, and wash vegetables.

Having these resources at your disposal will give you the confidence to attempt any recipe in this cookbook. While you don't have to buy every gadget on the market right first, upgrading to higher-quality versions of these necessities will greatly improve your cooking experience.

Elevating flavors are among the basic ingredients.

After discussing the tools, let's focus on the fundamental elements, which serve as the foundation for flavor. These elements, which are similar to the notes of a melody in the realm of simple cuisine, combine to make symphonious and gratifying dishes. Let's examine a few of these dependable food sources:

- **Olive oil:** A kitchen must-have is this multipurpose oil. Use it to roast, sauté, and dress salads. If you want the greatest flavor, choose extra virgin olive oil.

- **Herbs and Spices:** A dash of herbs and spices may transform an ordinary dish into something special. Basil,

thyme, oregano, garlic
powder, and paprika are
popular options.

- **Pepper and salt:** The basis
  of seasoning is these two
  essentials. For the most
  flavorful dishes, spend money
  on high-quality sea salt and
  freshly ground black pepper.

- **Garlic and onions:** Many
  savory meals are built on
  these aromatics. They give

your cooking more nuance and complexity.

- **Citrus Lemons, limes, and oranges** give savory and sweet foods a zesty freshness. The juice and zest can be added as a finishing touch or to marinades and sauces.

- **Vinegar:** Your dishes get more acidic and tangy when you use vinegar. Excellent options include balsamic, red wine, white wine, and apple cider vinegar.

- **Tomatoes in cans:** Tomatoes in cans are a pantry staple. They act as the foundation for a huge variety of sauces, soups, and stews.

- **Stock or Broth:** Stock or broth, whether made from beef, poultry, or vegetables, provides the tasty base for many savory recipes.

- **Grain products and legumes:** For robust and full meals, keep a variety of grains like rice, quinoa, and pasta on hand, along with canned or dried beans.

- **Maple syrup or honey:** The flavors of both sweet and savory foods can be harmoniously balanced using these natural sweeteners.

- **Tamari or soy sauce:** Use these to give your recipes a deeper umami flavor and a touch of saltiness.

- **Nuts and Seeds:** Almonds, walnuts, and seeds like sesame and pumpkin can give foods and salads a snap and a nutty flavor.

You can tackle a variety of dishes from "Skinnytaste Simple Cookbook" if you have these basic components in your home. These materials serve as the blank canvas for your culinary paintings. They are the undiscovered ingredients that will give your food depth, complexity, and that wonderful homemade flavor.

You'll see these components combined in unique and

delectable ways throughout this cookbook. We've carefully chosen recipes that demonstrate the magic of combining these culinary necessities to make delectable dishes while keeping things simple.

Keep in mind that cooking is a skill that can be developed with practice as I set off on this culinary adventure together. You may express your creativity while feeding yourself and your loved ones through this type of art. So, armed with these components and tools, let's explore "Skinnytaste Simple Cookbook"'s core principles.

You'll find a treasure mine of recipes that celebrate the elegance of simplicity in the kitchen in the pages that follow. I"ve created every recipe, from morning pleasures to one-pot wonders, with love and simplicity in mind. So take your apron, fasten it, and prepare to set off on a gastronomic journey that will alter the way you view cooking.

Good appetite!

"Skinnytaste Simple Cookbook" is more than simply a cookbook; it's a means to start eating more sensibly and healthily. The recipes in these pages are intended to demonstrate that making delectable, healthy meals doesn't require a lengthy list of ingredients or hours of your time. These recipes will make your life simpler while pleasing your palate, whether you're cooking for yourself, your family, or your friends.

You'll come across a variety of gastronomic treats as we progress through the book's chapters. Each meal is a testament to the power of simplicity, from tasty breakfasts that get your day going to mouthwatering dinners that make your evenings cozy.

This assortment has been thoughtfully chosen to satisfy a range of dietary choices and requirements. You can find recipes that suit your needs whether you're a vegetarian, a meat lover, or you're on a certain diet. Additionally, we've provided nutritional data for each meal so you can choose wisely and achieve your health objectives.

You can find useful advice and insights to help you maximize your time in the kitchen throughout "Skinnytaste Simple Cookbook." These pearls of knowledge will streamline your cooking process, making it even simpler and more pleasurable. They range from meal planning to effective prep practices.

Remember that the experience of cooking and dining with loved ones is what this cookbook is all about, not just the food. In a society that frequently values convenience over quality, it's about rediscovering the delight of nourishing, home-cooked cuisine.

So let's dig in and begin learning about the world of wholesome dishes with minimal ingredients. We'll set out on a journey together to make your kitchen a space for inspiration, nourishing food, and, most importantly, simplicity I appreciate you making

"Skinnytaste Simple Cookbook" your dining companion. Let's start a meal!

Chapter 1
Morning Delights

Imagine that your kitchen is bathed in a warm, golden glow as the sun peeks over the horizon. Freshly brewed coffee's aroma mixes with the alluring smells of toast with butter and sizzling bacon in the air. The image conjures up feelings of security, sustenance, and the hope of a fresh day. Undoubtedly, and with good cause, breakfast has a particular place in our hearts.

The Morning Routine

Breakfast is more than simply a meal; it's a ritual that provides a break from the rest of our busy days. It's our first opportunity to fill up after a night of rest and establish the tone for the day. However, many of us rush through our mornings in the busyness of modern life, grabbing a coffee to go or skipping breakfast entirely. We're here to rectify it since it's a lost chance.

Breakfast's significance cannot be emphasized. When you give your body a healthy breakfast, you give it the energy and nutrition it needs to start your metabolism and keep it alert and focused all day. According to numerous studies, people who regularly have a balanced breakfast are more likely to keep a healthy weight, make better food decisions throughout the day, and perform better at work or school.

The Breakfast Test

We know how chaotic mornings can be. Deadlines loom, the snooze button tempts, and getting the kids ready for school can seem like a marathon. We specifically created this chapter to assist you in easily overcoming the breakfast difficulty. The philosophy of "Skinnytaste Simple Cookbook" centers around living a simple life while nourishing your body, and it starts with breakfast.

You'll find a variety of morning treats in this chapter that are not only quick and simple to make but also wonderfully tasty and healthy. These recipes are divided into many categories so that there is something for every taste and dietary requirement. We have options for everyone, whether you want quick smoothies like to make breakfast the night before, or prefer a hot and filling start to your day.

Morning Fuel for Everyone

We understand that breakfast is a very individualized meal and that what works for one person might not work for another. Because of this, we've included a wide variety of dishes, each of which is designed for a particular type of breakfast. We have recipes that suit all lifestyles, whether you're a busy parent, an early riser with little time, or someone who enjoys a leisurely breakfast.

Do you typically start your day off quickly and with little time to spare? With this collection of quick and simple recipes, you can have a filling breakfast in no time. Our portable breakfasts are ideal for hectic mornings when you need something you can take with you. Perhaps you prefer on-the-go solutions.

I have included make-ahead options that can be prepared the night before for people who love the idea of a full breakfast but want to reduce morning prep. Just get up, get your breakfast out of the refrigerator, and enjoy. It guarantees that you won't ever skip breakfast again and is the ultimate time saver.

On the other hand, if you enjoy making food and taking your time in the mornings, our warm and filling breakfast recipes will tickle your taste buds. These delicacies, which range from fluffy omelets to luscious pancakes, are meant to be enjoyed when you have the time to take your time and enjoy each bite.

Showing You How to Create Breakfasts

You'll discover detailed directions as you look through the dishes in this chapter that make preparing your morning meal a snap. Each recipe has been carefully crafted to be understandable even to the most inexperienced cooks by being straightforward, succinct, and easy to follow. You can precisely estimate how long it will take to prepare your morning masterpiece because cooking times are provided.

I've also provided serving recommendations and styling advice so you may adapt each dish to your preferences. These minor adjustments, such as a drizzle of honey, a scattering of almonds, or a dash of your preferred spice, can transform your breakfast from ordinary to gourmet.

However, we are aware that words can only do so much to capture how exquisite these breakfast treats are. To help you get inspired, we've included gorgeous food photographs with each recipe. We want you to be able to see the eye-catching hues, alluring textures, and healthy components that go into each dish. Our intention is to get you enthusiastic about getting out of bed in the morning so you may create and enjoy these breakfast works of art.

So let's get right to the meat of our breakfast menu without further ado. "Skinnytaste Simple" has something unique in store for you, whether you're a devoted breakfast enthusiast or someone wishing to rekindle your love for the morning meal. Make breakfast the highlight of your day by donning an apron and getting hungry.

Blender Sensations

Let's begin our exploration of breakfast options with a category that is ideal for people who prefer to keep things simple and handy: smoothies. These liquid marvels seem to have been sent to us by the breakfast gods. They are quick to prepare, flexible, and highly nourishing.

Imagine a delicious concoction that combines the rich hues of ripe berries, the creamy texture of yogurt or nut milk, and the energizing zing of citrus. These smoothie sensations are not only a visual treat but also a flavor explosion that will enliven your morning and awaken your taste buds.

The smoothie recipes have you covered if you need an energy boost, a vitamin dose, or a protein-rich start to your day. You'll find options that match your taste and dietary requirements, from traditional combinations like the Berry Blast to exotic twists like the Tropical Paradise.

Night Oats: A Jar of Breakfast

You're in for a treat if you like hearty, filling breakfast items that you can grab and go. Our recipes for overnight oats are a revelation; they're a morning meal that can be prepared the night before and eaten as soon as you wake up.

Before going to bed, you can quickly put together a jar with oats, milk (or a dairy-free substitute), and your preferred toppings. The flavors combine while the oats soak overnight, absorbing the liquid and yielding a creamy, decadent breakfast.

The overnight oats recipes include anything from tried-and-true combos like chocolate and peanut butter to creative twists like the traditional cinnamon and apple. What's best? With the addition of your preferred fruits, nuts, seeds, and sweeteners, you may customize them to your heart's desire.

Quick Egg Dishes: Perfectly Protein-Packed!

The quick egg recipes will have you eagerly hopping out of bed if you enjoy the savory side of breakfast. With their abundance of protein and other vital minerals, eggs are a nutritional powerhouse. They are also highly adaptable, enabling you to quickly prepare a filling breakfast.

The recipes cover the whole range of egg-based delights, from fluffy scrambled eggs to perfectly poached delicacies. We have the ideal dish for you, whether you're craving a traditional omelet, a frittata packed with vegetables, or a breakfast sandwich that hits all the right notes.

Our egg dishes are made to make preparing eggs in the morning simple. Whether you prefer your eggs firm and fully cooked or soft and runny, we provide you step-by-step directions for attaining the ideal flavor and texture. Additionally, you may alter up your daily routine and never grow tired of breakfast thanks to the variety of component combinations.

Fuel Your Morning Effortlessly

The underlying philosophy for these breakfast recipes is simplicity, as you'll discover as you look through them. No matter how you want to eat breakfast or what time you get up in the morning, we want to make sure you have access to healthy food options.

Making breakfast is something we want to be fun, stress-free, and, most importantly, rewarding. With a variety of dishes that suit various schedules and palates, you can reclaim your morning meal and get your day off to a good start.

So, enjoy breakfast's simplicity. Enjoy the pleasure of waking up to these delicious dishes that will nourish your body, tempt your taste senses, and set the mood for a good day. As you peruse our breakfast offerings, keep in mind that breakfast is more than simply a meal; it's a chance to energize yourself, take pleasure in a peaceful time, and appreciate the little things in life.

With the correct recipes at your disposal, breakfast won't be a problem for you anymore; instead, it'll be a wonderful morning routine. So without further ado, let's go off on a breakfast adventure that honors the wonder of simplicity and the satisfaction of beginning your day with a filling, healthy meal.

Berries & Blast Smoothie

Ingredients

- 1 cup of mixed berries (strawberries, blueberries, and raspberries), fresh or frozen
a single ripe banana
- 1/2 cup Greek yogurt (or yogurt without dairy)
- 1/2 cup almond milk (or any other type of milk you want)

- 1 tablespoon of optionally additional honey for sweetness
- Ice cubes (optional; for a cooler smoothie)

Instructions

1. Combine the Greek yogurt, ripe banana, almond milk, and honey (if using) in a blender.
2. You can add a few ice cubes to the blender for a cooler smoothie if you'd like.

3. Make sure there are no lumps and blend all the ingredients until they are smooth and creamy.

4. Taste the smoothie and, if necessary, add additional honey to balance the sweetness.

5. Transfer the Berry Blast Smoothie to a glass, if desired, decorate with a few fresh berries, and savor!

Cooking time is five minutes.

Serving Advice

- To make your Berry Blast Smoothie even more refreshing, serve it in a chilled glass.
- Top with some granola or chia seeds for texture and extra nutrition.

Oats with Chocolate Peanut Butter Leftovers

Ingredients

- 1 tablespoon chocolate powder - 1/2 cup rolled oats

- 1 tablespoon maple syrup or honey
- 1 teaspoon of peanut butter
- 1/2 cup almond milk (or any other type of milk you want)
- 1/2 ripe banana, mashed

Add a dash of salt, a half teaspoon of vanilla flavor, and 1 tablespoon of chopped peanuts as a garnish.

- 1 tablespoon of miniature chocolate chips (optional, as a garnish)

Instructions

1. Combine the rolled oats, cocoa powder, honey or maple syrup, peanut butter, almond milk, mashed banana, salt, and vanilla extract in a mason jar or other airtight container.

2. Combine all the ingredients by thoroughly stirring them together.

3. To help the oats soak up the liquid and flavors, cover the jar or container and place it in the refrigerator overnight (or for at least 4 hours).

4. Stir the oats thoroughly in the morning. You can thin out the mixture if it is too thick by adding a little more almond milk.

5. Add chopped peanuts and micro chocolate chips to the top of your chocolate peanut butter overnight oats, if you want.

6. Eat your meal straight from the jar or, if you'd rather, transfer it to a bowl.

5 minutes of preparation time (including overnight refrigeration)*

You can make these oats ahead of time for a few days if you're in a rush, giving you a simple and filling breakfast alternative for the rest of the week.

Breakfast Quesadilla with Spinach and Feta

Ingredients

- 4 huge eggs

- 2 large whole wheat tortillas

- A single cup of new, newborn spinach leaves

- 1/2 cup feta cheese crumbles

- Salt & pepper to taste

- Cooking spray or a little amount of olive oil.

Instructions

1. Beat the eggs in a bowl, then season with salt and pepper to taste.

2. Lightly coat a non-stick skillet with cooking spray or a small quantity of olive oil and heat it over medium heat.

3. Add half of the beaten eggs to the skillet and lay them out

equally. Cook the eggs for 1-2 minutes, or until they start to set.

4. Top the eggs in the skillet with a whole wheat tortilla.

5. Quickly and evenly distribute half of the feta cheese crumbles and half of the baby spinach leaves over the tortilla.

6. Carefully fold the remaining tortilla half over the toppings to form a quesadilla.

7. Continue cooking for an additional 1 to 2 minutes, or until

the cheese is melted and the bottom is brown.

8. When the quesadilla is golden brown and the eggs are done, carefully flip it over to cook the other side.

9. After removing the first quesadilla from the skillet, prepare the second one using the remaining components.

10. To serve hot, cut each quesadilla into wedges.

15 minutes for cooking

Serve your spinach and feta breakfast quesadilla with a side of fresh salsa or a dollop of Greek yogurt for a little extra flavor.

The gastronomic delights you will have in the morning don't end with these breakfast dishes. They're made to be immensely gratifying, quick, and easy, making sure that your day gets off to the ideal start.

Whether you choose the zingy Berry Blast Smoothie, the time-saving Chocolate Peanut Butter Overnight Oats, or the hearty Spinach and Feta Breakfast Quesadilla, every meal offers a delicious way to fuel your body and get you ready for the day.

So enjoy the pleasure of a healthy breakfast. It's a simple yet effective method to put self-care first, increase your energy, and give your daily routine a healthy jumpstart. With these dishes at your disposal, breakfast won't seem like a challenge anymore but rather a chance to enjoy easy, delectable moments that will brighten your day. Have a great breakfast and may it be the first of many fantastic breakfast adventures!

Options for breakfast on the go

Breakfast burrito

Ingredients

- Black beans

- Salsa

- Scrambled eggs

- Whole wheat tortilla

 - Chopped bell peppers

- Optional cheese crumbles

Instructions

1. Make scrambled eggs with the vegetables and seasonings of your choice.

2. Use a microwave or a skillet to reheat the tortilla.

3. Arrange the tortilla with scrambled eggs, salsa, black beans, and cheese (if preferred).

4. Once you've rolled it up, your breakfast burrito is prepared.

Chia Pudding Left Over

Ingredients

the Chia seed

- Greek yogurt (or yogurt without dairy)

- Milk (or milk substitute)

- Maple or honey syrup

- Fresh fruit (such as sliced bananas and berries)

Instructions

1. In a jar or other container, combine the chia seeds, yogurt, milk, and sweetener.

2. Keep it chilled for the night.

3. When you add fresh fruit on top in the morning, you have a portable chia pudding.

Muffins for breakfast

Ingredients

Whole-wheat muffins

- Cooked bacon or turkey sausage

- Scrambled eggs

- Cheese slices

Instructions

1. Fill a whole wheat muffin with scrambled eggs, cooked bacon or turkey sausage, and a slice of cheese.

2. To make breakfast you can take and go, wrap it in foil or parchment paper.

Yogurt Parfait

Ingredients

- Greek yogurt (or yogurt without dairy)
- Fruit, fresh or frozen - Granola
- Maple or honey syrup

Instructions

1. Arrange fruit, granola, and yogurt in a carry-on container.
2. Drizzle with maple syrup or honey.
3. Put the lid on the container, and your yogurt parfait is prepared for travel.

A sandwich with peanut butter and banana

Ingredients

- Wraps or whole-wheat bread

- Banana slices - Peanut butter (or almond butter)

- Honey, if desired

Instructions

1. Butter the bread or wrap it with peanut butter.

2. If preferred, include sliced banana and a sprinkle of honey.

3. To make it into a portable breakfast, fold, roll, and wrap it in foil or plastic wrap.

These wholesome, on-the-go breakfast options are excellent for those hectic mornings when you need to bring breakfast with you. Even while you're on the go, you may have a healthy lunch by customizing them.

Chapter 2

Snacks and Appetizers

Consider yourself the host of a gathering of friends or relatives. As everyone interacts and catches up, laughter permeates the room. But what is the secret ingredient that makes the experience better? The enticing aroma of your guests' appetizers and snacks is what draws them in and begins the culinary journey.

The Function of Starters and Snacks

The unsung heroes of each event are the snacks and appetizers. They are essential for establishing the ambiance, titillating the palate, and staving off hunger while the main meal is cooking. Beyond being useful, these little miracles are a testament to the pleasure of eating and entertaining with food. Appetizers and snacks act as fillers in the context of a balanced diet. They can provide you with food and energy, refueling you during hectic days or reviving you after exercise. However, they serve as more than just a source of energy and provide a chance to savor delicious flavors, textures, and combinations.

The Benefits of Pairing

In the world of appetizers and snacks, pairing is a skill. It's the alchemy of combining flavors and textures to produce a mouthwatering symphony of flavor. The ideal appetizer or snack can improve your overall dining experience, whether you're sipping wine, a craft brew, or a cup of tea.

You'll find a great selection of dishes divided into three categories in this chapter: "Finger Foods," "Dips and Spreads," and "Healthier Chip Alternatives." There is something for every occasion, from informal get-togethers to formal soirées, as each segment gives a distinctive viewpoint on the world of appetizers and nibbles.

Delightful Bite-Sized Finger Foods

The main event is the finger snacks. These bite-sized, tasty nibbles are made to be enjoyed easily with one hand, which makes them ideal for mingling and conversation. They are the first items on the appetizer tray to disappear, leaving visitors excitedly requesting more.

Capital Skewers

Ingredients

- Wooden skewers
- Cherry tomatoes
- Fresh mozzarella balls
- Fresh basil leaves
- Balsamic glaze

Instructions

1. Wrap a fresh basil leaf, a little mozzarella ball, and a cherry tomato around each wooden skewer.

2. Add a glaze of balsamic vinegar.

3. Put the skewers on a serving platter and proceed to serve.

Suggestions for Pairing: Caprese skewers go well with a refreshing Sauvignon Blanc. The fresh tastes of the tomatoes and basil are enhanced by the wine's acidity.

Dates wrapped in bacon

Ingredients

- Pitted Medjool dates
- Whole almonds
- Slices of bacon

Instructions

1. Set the oven's temperature to 375°F (190°C).
2. Place a whole nut inside each date that has been pitted.

3. Wrap a piece of bacon around each date and fasten it with a toothpick.

4. Set the individually wrapped dates on a baking pan.

5. Bake the bacon for 15 to 20 minutes, or until crispy.

6. Present hot.

Suggestions for Pairing: These savory and sweet delicacies go perfectly with a drink of champagne or sparkling wine.

Between bites, the bubbles will clear your palate.

Flavorful Companions: Dips and Spreads

The social butterflies of the appetizer world are dips and spreads. They encourage social interaction and group dipping and sharing. These toppings, which range from fiery salsa to creamy hummus, may elevate common snacks to amazing levels.

Guacamole

Ingredients

- Finished avocados

- Finely chopped red onion -
Chopped fresh cilantro

- Minced jalapenos (modified to
taste)

Citrus juice

- Tortilla chips for dipping - Salt
and pepper to taste

Instructions

1. Use a fork to mash several ripe
avocados in a bowl.

2. Add the lime juice, minced jalapenos, cilantro, and red onion that has been chopped.

3. To taste, add salt and pepper to the dish.

4. Present alongside tortilla chips.

Suggestions for Pairing:
Guacamole's creamy richness and a crisp Mexican lager go well beautifully. The texture of the avocado enhances the crispness of the beer.

Traditional hummus

Ingredients

- Cooked or canned chickpeas; - Tahini; - Lemon juice

- Ground cumin - Ground garlic - Olive oil - Paprika

- Vegetable sticks or pita bread for dipping

Instructions

1. Process the chickpeas, tahini, lemon juice, garlic, extra virgin olive oil, ground cumin, and salt in a food processor until smooth.

2. Taste the dish, then season as necessary.

3. Transfer to a serving bowl, top with paprika, and drizzle with olive oil.

4. Offer pita bread or vegetable sticks with the meal.

Suggestions for Pairing Hummus pairs well with a glass of dry white wine, such as Chardonnay, because of its earthy taste. The acidity of the wine balances the hummus's lemony flavor.

Alternatives to Healthy Chips: Crunchy Satisfaction

Chips are irresistibly alluring, but there is some concern about how they may affect your health. Healthy chip substitutes can help in this situation. These snacks satisfy your need for crunch and flavor without sacrificing your health.

Sweet potatoes chips

Ingredients

- Thinly sliced sweet potatoes -
Olive oil

- To taste, salt and pepper

Instructions

1. Set the oven's temperature to 375°F (190°C).

2. In a bowl, mix the sweet potatoes that have been thinly sliced with the olive oil, salt, and pepper.

3. On a baking sheet, arrange the sweet potato slices in a single layer.

4. Bake for 15-20 minutes, or until crisp and just browned.

5. Permit cooling before serving.

Suggestions for Pairing: The natural sweetness of sweet potato chips complements a glass of citrus-infused sparkling water perfectly. The two together are revitalizing and guilt-free.

kettle chips

Ingredients

Fresh kale leaves with the stems cut off and broken into little pieces. Olive oil. Salt and your preferred seasonings (such as chili flakes, nutritional yeast, or garlic powder).

Instructions

1. Set the oven's temperature to 300°F (150°C).

2. Apply olive oil to the torn kale leaves and massage them to distribute it evenly.

3. Add salt and your preferred seasonings.

4. Spread out the kale pieces in a single layer on a baking pan.

5. Bake for 10 to 15 minutes, or until crisp but not burned.

6. Wait until they are cool before serving.

Suggestions for Pairing: A revitalizing green smoothie goes perfectly with kale chips. The crunch comes from the chips, while the colorful flavors and vitamins come from the smoothie. It's a vibrant pair that's wholesome and gratifying.

Investigating the World of Snacks and Appetizers

A wealth of culinary innovation may be found in the area of appetizers and snacks. It's a place where tastes meld together, textures jive, and the joy of sharing food draws people together. You've only seen a small portion of the options here; there are countless more that are just waiting to be discovered.

The ideal starter or snack may take your gathering to new heights, whether you're organizing a casual game night with friends, a family picnic in the park, or a sophisticated cocktail party. You may make a spread that not only fulfills your appetites but also enthralls your guests with a little imagination and inspiration.

Always keep in mind that these recipes are just launching points as you go out on your adventures with appetizers and snacks. You are allowed to explore, alter, and add your personal touches. After all, these culinary pleasures' appeal resides in their adaptation to your taste and diversity.

The Senses Captivated: Food Photography

It's not just about flavor and feel when it comes to properly appreciating the world of appetizers and snacks; it's also about the visual feast. Your culinary adventure is greatly inspired by food photography. The experience is enhanced by the striking hues, alluring textures, and creative presentation.

Try to picture the bright reds of freshly created salsa, the crispiness of sweet potato chips, or the rich, creamy greens of a well-made guacamole. Your senses are roused by these images, which also cause your mouth to wet and your interest in food to soar.

Snacks and appetizers are more than simply food; they're a call to engage, discover, and appreciate the small pleasures of life. Each meal is a special occasion, whether you're savoring a luscious bacon-wrapped date, dipping pita bread into creamy hummus, or enjoying the crunch of kale chips.

So keep in mind that these recipes are designed to make your life easier, more flavorful, and more fun as you begin your culinary journey through the world of appetizers and snacks. May these foods please your palate and make you happy, whether you're serving them to visitors or just enjoying a lonely snack time.

You are not only nourishing your body with each bite but also your spirit. You're honoring the beauty of simplicity, the joys of sharing, and the joy of flavor. So gather your ingredients, put on your apron, and let's go on an adventure into the world of appetizers and nibbles.

I appreciate you selecting "Skinnytaste Simple Cookbook" as your gastronomic ally. The journey has begun!

Chapter 3

Quick Lunches to Quench Your Midday Craving

The beautiful midday period that connects breakfast and dinner is lunchtime. When hunger strikes, we seek food that would not only satisfy our stomachs but also satisfy our taste buds. Beyond simply quelling our appetite, a filling and wholesome lunch nourishes both body and mind, enabling us to take on the rest of the day's activities.

The Influence of Lunch

Our daily routine is not complete without lunch, which is essential to our general well-being. It's the meal that restores our energy, sharpens our focus, and gives us the nutrition we need for the highest degree of production. A healthy lifestyle's foundation is built on a well-balanced meal, which is more than just a noon ritual.

Imagine your workday: a hectic schedule, an active office, or a number of things vying for your attention. It's simple to get lost in the commotion and forget how important lunch is. The truth is that a filling lunch can make your day better. It can lift your spirits, sharpen your brain, and give you the energy and clarity you need to face obstacles.

Lunchtime bliss with balanced meals

Balance is essential when creating the ideal lunch. A well-rounded lunch includes foods from different dietary categories, ensuring that you get a range of important nutrients. The components of a balanced meal are listed below:

1. Lean Protein: Protein keeps you full, fuels your muscles, and promotes development and repair. Excellent sources of protein include options like fish, beans, chicken, turkey, tofu, and other meats.

2. Healthy Carbohydrates: Your body uses carbohydrates as its main fuel. To give enduring energy, choose complex carbohydrates like whole grains, quinoa, brown rice, or whole-grain bread.

3. Fiber-Rich Vegetables: Vegetables are rich in fiber, vitamins, and minerals that promote healthy digestion. Carrots, bell peppers, broccoli, and leafy greens are all excellent options.

4. Healthy Fats: Healthy fats are necessary for optimal brain and general health. Include ingredients in your meal such as avocado, olive oil, almonds, and seeds.

5. Portion management: Portion management is just as vital as balancing. Be mindful of portion amounts to avoid overeating.

Various Ideas for Quick Lunches

After discussing the importance of lunch and the elements of a balanced meal, let's explore some short lunch options that satisfy your appetite while still meeting all the nutritional requirements. These recipes range from colorful salads to filling wraps to delectable sandwiches, all of which are meant to make your lunchtime a treat.

Quinoa salad from the Mediterranean

Ingredients

- Cooked quinoa
- Halved cherry tomatoes

- Diced cucumber

- Finely chopped red onion

- Pitted and sliced Kalamata olives

- Crumbled feta cheese

- Chopped fresh parsley

- Olive oil

Citrus juice

- To taste, salt and pepper

Instructions

1. Combine cooked quinoa,
Kalamata olives, cucumber, red
onion, and crumbled feta cheese
in a big bowl.

2. Garnish with lemon juice and olive oil. Add salt and pepper to taste.

3. Combine everything by tossing it all together.

4. Add fresh parsley as a garnish and serve.

Relationship Suggestion: A glass of refreshing Sauvignon Blanc goes perfectly with this Mediterranean quinoa salad. The acidity of the wine enhances the salad's freshness.

Chipotle Avocado Wrap

Ingredients

- Sliced grilled chicken breast

- Sliced avocado

- Mixture of greens

- Tortillas made with whole grains

- Greek yogurt (as a nutritious substitute for mayo)

- Mustard from Dijon

- To taste, salt and pepper

Instructions:

1. To make a tasty spread, combine Greek yogurt and Dijon mustard in a small bowl. Add salt and pepper to taste.

2. Place the yogurt-mustard mixture on a whole-grain tortilla wrap.

3. Arrange grilled chicken slices, avocado, and mixed greens on top.

4. Fold the tortilla's sides in and securely roll it up.

5. To serve, split the wrap in half.

Relationship Suggestion: The flavors of the Chicken Avocado Wrap match perfectly with an iced green tea for a delicious lunch.

The Caprese Panini

Ingredients

Whole-grain or Ciabatta bread; fresh mozzarella slices

- Sliced tomatoes

Olive oil (for grilling), balsamic glaze, and fresh basil leaves

Instructions

1. Sandwich pieces of ciabatta or whole-grain bread between slices of fresh mozzarella, tomato, and basil.

2. Spread some olive oil and balsamic glaze on the inside of the bread.

3. Set a skillet or a panini press to medium heat.

4. Grill the sandwich until the cheese has melted and the bread has become crispy.

5. Cut and present.

Relationship Suggestion: The aromas of the Caprese Panini are complemented by a light and fruity Pinot Noir, making for a lovely pairing.

Lunch on the Run: Simple Pleasures

Fresh and vibrant salads

For those looking for a healthy, light lunch, salads are a lunchtime favorite. They are adaptable, enabling you to experiment with different ingredients and dressings to produce a dish that is flavorful.

Traditional Cobb salad

Ingredients

- Diced grilled chicken breast
- Chopped romaine lettuce
- Sliced hard-boiled eggs
- Halved cherry tomatoes
- Diced avocado
- Blue cheese in crumbles
- Bacon crumbs

- Dressing with balsamic vinaigrette

Instructions

1. Arrange a bed of chopped Romaine lettuce in a big basin.

2. Top with chopped grilled chicken, hard-boiled eggs, cherry tomatoes, avocado, blue cheese crumbles, and bacon bits.

3. Add a balsamic vinaigrette dressing drizzle.

4. Your Classic Cobb Salad is ready to serve; gently toss to blend.

Relationship Suggestion: A mild Pinot Grigio or an iced tea goes perfectly with the Cobb Salad's bold ingredients.

Sandwiches are a traditional option.

Sandwiches are a classic lunch option that are loved for their ease and practicality. They are ideal for people seeking a filling and portable lunch.

Sandwich with turkey and cranberries

Ingredients

turkey breast cut into slices with cranberry sauce

- Small spinach leaves - Slices of whole-grain bread

Instructions

Two pieces of whole-grain bread should be spread out.

2. Arrange cranberry sauce, baby spinach leaves, and thinly sliced turkey breast in one piece.

3. To finish off your Turkey and Cranberry Sandwich, place the second slice of bread on top.

4. Now that it has been cut in half diagonally, you may enjoy it.

Relationship Suggestion: The Turkey and Cranberry Sandwich pairs well with a cool glass of sparkling water with a squeeze of lime.

Upgrade Your Lunch Experience

There are many delicious options for quick and filling meals, including salads and sandwiches. These recipes are made to make lunchtime a breeze, whether you prefer the crispness of a Classic Cobb Salad or the cozy simplicity of a Turkey and Cranberry Sandwich.

They make sure you stay energized and focused throughout the day with their well-balanced blend of flavors and nutrients. Therefore, when you consider these lunch options, keep in mind that you have the ability to improve your lunchtime experience and appreciate each meal.

These simple, flavorful, and nourishing quick lunch ideas are more than just meals; they're a celebration of all three. They provide you with the energy and satiety you need to take on the remainder of your day since they contain the ideal ratio of protein, carbs, healthy fats, and fresh vegetables.

Do not forget that lunchtime is a time for self-care and recharging, not just a break in your daily schedule. Every bite is a chance to put your health first and appreciate the delights of healthy cuisine, whether you're savoring a Caprese Panini, relishing a Chicken Avocado Wrap, or enjoying a Mediterranean Quinoa Salad.

Variety to Satisfy All Palates

The variety of these quick lunch options is what makes them so appealing. They satisfy a wide range of palates, nutritional requirements, and culinary preferences. There is a recipe here that will appeal to your palate, whether you enjoy the colorful tastes of the Mediterranean, lean protein, or traditional Caprese dishes.

These lunches are also ideal for people who are often on the go. These dishes are made to be tasty and practical whether you're working from home, at the office, or simply taking it easy outside. Busy professionals, students, or anyone who values a healthy lunch in the middle of a busy day will find them to be the perfect companions.

Nutrition and portion control must be balanced.

While flavor is important, it's critical to keep in mind the value of balance in your meal. These recipes have all been thoughtfully created to offer a blend of necessary nutrients, ensuring that you receive the energy, vitamins, and minerals you require. To avoid overeating, though, it's crucial to use portion control.

Be mindful of the suggested serving sizes for each ingredient as you put together your lunch. This not only enables you to keep a healthy calorie intake but also lets you fully appreciate the flavors without leaving you feeling stuffed or lethargic.

Additionally, it's crucial to pay attention to your body's hunger signals. Eat until you're pleasantly full, not until you're stuffed to the gills. Keep in mind that lunch should make you feel energized, not sluggish.

The art of enjoying the little things.

It's simple to overlook the simple pleasures of lunch in the hustle and bustle of daily life. But a delicious meal can bring joy, serenity, and a gentle reminder that feeding yourself is a form of self-care. These lunches are an invitation to savor the present, whether you're eating a vibrant salad, a filling wrap, or a toasty panini.

Don't go for a hasty snack or a subpar dinner the next time you get a noon hunger pang. Take time for yourself, practice the art of simple pleasures, and treat yourself to a fast meal that will nourish your body and elevate your spirits.

You have the ability to make your lunchtime a celebration of flavor, balance, and self-care with these recipes at your disposal. So gather your ingredients, make these delicious dishes, and enjoy the pleasure of an easy lunch that satisfies both the body and the soul.

Remember that these recipes are just the beginning of your culinary journey as you delve into the world of quick lunches. They're here to encourage you, to stoke your imagination, and to serve as a reminder that even the most straightforward meal can be a work of art.

May these recipes serve as a reminder that wholesome food can be a source of solace, joy, and connection, whether you're preparing lunch for yourself, sharing it with loved ones, or taking a quiet moment to yourself. You aren't just nourishing your body with each bite; you are also savoring the little pleasures in life.

I appreciate your participation in my culinary exploration of the world of quick lunches. Be guided by your taste buds, and may every meal be a celebration of delicacy and health. Make the most of your opportunity to shine during lunch.

Chapter 4

Easy Dinners: Overcoming the Weeknight Dinner Conundrum

Weeknights can be a flurry of frantic activities. We may feel exhausted and pushed for time as a result of work, school, errands, and other commitments. The thought of cooking a handmade meal could seem like an impossible task. However, there is a treasure trove of recipes created especially for hectic evenings in the realm of culinary delights. This investigation into hassle-free dinners will focus on quick and delectable main dishes that not only save you time but also please your palate. These recipes are your go-to tools for solving the weeknight supper conundrum, from sizzling stir-fries to one-pan miracles and hearty skillet entrees.

The Challenge of Weeknight Dinners

Imagine this: You've just returned from a busy day at work on a Tuesday evening. You need to finish some home chores, the kids have soccer practice, and you want a meal that's not only quick to prepare but also satisfying and tasty. There is urgency to prepare dinner because time is running out.

Many people are familiar with the difficulty of preparing a weeknight meal. It's about finding a method to strike a balance between the necessity of a home-cooked meal and the rigors of daily living. It's about finding a solution to the dilemma of how to create a filling meal without spending hours in the kitchen. Thankfully, we have a solution in the form of easy-to-prepare main dishes that can be prepared on weeknights.

Quick and Delicious Main Dishes

Let's get started with the main meals that will transform your weeknight dinners as we continue on our culinary adventure. These dishes focus on flavorful ingredients and bright tastes for your evening meal, not just quickness.

Stir-fried chicken and vegetables

Ingredients

- Bell peppers, broccoli, carrots chopped assorted veggies
- Boneless, skinless chicken breasts, thinly sliced
- Minced garlic cloves
- Minced ginger
- Tobacco sauce
- Sesame seed oil
- corn starch
- Serving options: rice or noodles

Instructions

1. To make a sauce, combine soy sauce, sesame oil, and cornstarch in a bowl.

2. Set a wok or skillet over high heat.

3. Add a little oil and stir-fry the chicken slices until they are fully done. Take out of the skillet.

4. Stir-fry the minced garlic and ginger in the same skillet until fragrant, using additional oil if necessary.

5. Include the chopped vegetables and stir-fry them for a further few minutes, or until they're crisp and tender.

6. Add the cooked chicken back to the skillet, cover with sauce, and stir-fry for a couple of minutes.

7. Put rice or noodles on the table with the chicken and vegetable stir-fry.

Relationship Suggestion: The flavors of the Chicken and Vegetable Stir-Fry are enhanced by a glass of light, crisp Pinot Grigio, making it an excellent supper choice.

Salmon and vegetables in a sheet pan with lemon and herbs

Ingredients

- Salmon fillets
- A variety of veggies (zucchini, asparagus, cherry tomatoes)
- Slices of fresh lemon
- Fresh herbs (dill, thyme, or rosemary)

- Oil of olives

- Minced garlic

- To taste, salt and pepper

Instructions

1. Set the oven's temperature to 400°F (200°C).

2. Use parchment paper to line a sheet pan.

3. Arrange various vegetables and salmon fillets on the sheet pan.

4. Add salt and pepper and drizzle with olive oil before scattering with chopped garlic.

154

5. Scatter some herbs and lemon slices over top.

6. Roast the salmon in the oven for 15 to 20 minutes, or until it is cooked to your preference.

7. Directly off the sheet pan, serve the salmon and vegetables with lemon and herbs.

Relationship Suggestion: The rich flavors of the salmon and the zingy herb dressing are enhanced by a cool glass of Chardonnay.

Dietary Needs Adaptation

These dishes are adaptable to a variety of dietary requirements. Here are a few simple changes:

- **Vegetarian/Vegan Option:** To make the stir-fry vegetarian or vegan, swap the chicken for tofu or tempeh. Substitute plant-based seafood for the fish in the salmon sheet pan dish and increase the amount of vegetables instead.

- **Gluten-Free:** Make sure the noodles, rice, or other grains you choose are free of the protein gluten, and use gluten-free soy sauce in the stir-fry.

- **Low-Carb/Keto:** Leave out the noodles or swap them out for cauliflower rice in the stir-fry recipe. Choose low-carb vegetables like broccoli and cauliflower for the salmon on a sheet pan.

- **Dairy-Free:** These recipes are naturally free of dairy, but use caution when using sauces or condiments from the store as they might contain dairy ingredients.

Learning to Make Effortless Dinners

The goal of effortless meals is to master the chaos of weekday cooking while appreciating the satisfaction of a home-cooked meal. With the help of these recipes, you may turn a hectic evening into a leisurely mealtime. They serve as proof that making delectable and gratifying food doesn't require a culinary degree or a lot of time in the kitchen.

Remember that these recipes are your allies as you set out on your weeknight dinner adventures and fight the dinner conundrum. They're here to simplify your life, improve the flavor of your food, and brighten your evenings. So embrace weeknight cooking's simplicity, up the ante on your dinners, and enjoy the simple pleasure of a delicious meal shared with loved ones.

These simple dinners are just the start of your culinary adventure because the world of cooking is a wide panorama of flavors and options. They are here to encourage you, pique your imagination, and serve as a reminder that even on the busiest of days, delicious cuisine can be a source of solace and camaraderie.

I appreciate your participation in this culinary journey as we explore quick and delectable main dishes for hectic weeknight dinners. In addition to providing nourishment for your body, each meal you prepare fosters joy and community. So gather your ingredients, appreciate how straightforward these recipes are, and start enjoying the magic of weeknight cooking. savor each bite!

Chapter 5

One-Pot Wonders: Easier Meals with Less Cleanup

There is a magic spell that changes the way we prepare meals and clean up afterward in the world of culinary magic. One-pot cooking is a game-changer for time-constrained home cooks. Imagine cooking a big, tasty supper with just one pot or pan. There aren't any piles of filthy dishes or time-consuming cleanups; just pure convenience and deliciousness. In this investigation of one-pot marvels, we'll learn the technique of cooking quickly while sharing recipes that only call for one pot or pan and are suitable for both vegetarians and meat eaters.

One-Pot Cooking's Allure

Unravel the charm of one-pot cooking to start. It's a cooking method that promises ease of use, effectiveness, and flavor. But why is it so tempting, and why should it be in your arsenal of recipes?

Convenience personified

Consider the following case: After a long day at work, you arrive home ravenous and eager to prepare a filling lunch. After cooking, the prospect of dealing with a pile of dishes is intimidating. One-pot wonders come to the rescue in this situation. You won't have to worry about cleaning up after supper when you only have one pot or pan to do it in. It personifies convenience at its finest.

Time-Saving Magic

One-pot cooking recognizes that time is a valuable resource. The preparation and cleanup time are greatly decreased by reducing the amount of cookware and utensils. As a result, you'll spend more time interacting with your loved ones, spend less time cleaning dishes, and prepare dinner quickly.

Flavorful Harmony

One-pot meals should have flavor as well as convenience. Ingredients have the chance to combine and integrate their flavors when cooked in a single pot or pan, producing dishes that are flavorful, mellow, and brimming with richness. Each bite is like a musical composition of flavors.

One-Pot Wonders with Meat

168

With some delicious meat-based meals that will tickle your taste buds and streamline your dinner routine, let's explore the world of one-pot miracles.

Grilled Beef Stroganoff

Ingredients

- Ground beef - Finely chopped onion

- Minced garlic

- sliced mushrooms

- Sour cream

- Beef broth

– Paprika

- Noodles in egg

- Freshly chopped parsley (for garnish), with salt and pepper to taste

Instructions

1. Over medium-high heat, cook the ground beef in a big skillet.

2. Include sliced mushrooms, minced garlic, and diced onion. Sauté the vegetables until they are soft.

3. Add salt, pepper, and paprika.

4. Add beef broth and boil the mixture.

5. Include the egg noodles and cook them until they are soft and have absorbed the majority of the liquid.

6. Add sour cream and stir until the sauce becomes creamy.

7. Add fresh parsley as a garnish and serve.

Relationship Suggestion: The hearty and delicious flavors of the

Beef Stroganoff Skillet pair well with a glass of Merlot.

Delicious vegetarian one-pot meals

Here are some one-pot miracles that highlight the beauty of ingredients from plants for our vegetarian friends.

Risotto with spinach and mushrooms in one pot
Ingredients

rice, Arborio, and fresh spinach

sliced mushrooms

Finely sliced onion; vegetable

broth; and, if desired, white wine

- Parmesan cheese (or a vegan

substitute)

- Minced garlic

- Oil of olives

- To taste, salt and pepper

Instructions

1. Melt olive oil in a sizable skillet

or pot over medium heat.

2. Include sliced mushrooms, minced garlic, and diced onion. Sauté the mushrooms until they are soft.

3. Add the Arborio rice and stir. Cook for a few minutes, or until the rice is just starting to toast.

4. If wine is being used, add a splash and let it absorb.

5. Add vegetable broth gradually, one ladle at a time, stirring after each addition to ensure that the liquid is fully absorbed.

6. Stir in fresh spinach until it is wilted when the rice is creamy and cooked to your preferred level of doneness.

7. Add grated Parmesan cheese (or a vegan substitute) and stir.

8. Add salt and pepper, and then serve.

Relationship Suggestion:
Spinach and mushroom risotto's creamy consistency and earthy taste pair well with a crisp, fragrant Sauvignon Blanc.

One-Pot Magic for Everyone

One-pot cooking has benefits for everyone, whether you love meat or are a dedicated vegetarian. It's a culinary journey that makes life easier while improving the dinner-eating experience. The purpose of these recipes is to enjoy the pleasure of a home-cooked meal without the effort of cleanup, not only to make life easier.

Adjustment for Dietary Needs

Due to its adaptability, one-pot marvels can be made to meet a variety of dietary requirements and preferences. Here are some modifications you can make to these dishes to satisfy particular dietary needs:

Variations for vegetarians and vegans:

For a vegetarian version of the Beef Stroganoff Skillet, swap the ground beef for plant-based ground meat or crumbled tofu.
- Substitute vegan sour cream for sour cream made from dairy.
- If you want to make it vegan-friendly, use eggless noodles.

For the spinach and mushroom risotto in one pot:
- To make a recipe entirely vegetarian, swap out the chicken stock for veggie broth.

- To make a vegan version of Parmesan cheese, use nutritional yeast for regular cheese.

Gluten-Free Choices:

Make sure the rice or noodles you use are gluten-free for both recipes.
If necessary, substitute gluten-free vegetable broth.

Low-Carb/Keto-Friendly Modifications

- Serve the beef stroganoff over cauliflower rice or zucchini noodles instead of egg noodles when making the beef stroganoff skillet.

For the spinach and mushroom risotto in one pot

- To add a low-carb twist, swap out the Arborio rice for cauliflower rice.

- Change the amount of vegetable broth as necessary to reach the appropriate consistency.

Dairy-free substitutes include

For both recipes: - Substitute acceptable dairy-free sour cream or cheese in place of the dairy-based versions.

Like a culinary magic trick, one-pot cooking makes your life easier without sacrificing flavor. These dishes are proof that you can eat well and feel satisfied without having to deal with a messy kitchen. One-pot wonders have something for everyone, whether you favor meat-based recipes like the Beef Stroganoff Skillet or the vegetarian allure of the Spinach and Mushroom Risotto.

You'll experience a new level of joy in the kitchen as you learn to appreciate the simplicity and flavor of one-pot cooking. Instead of being constrained by pots and pans, the goal is to cherish the time spent with your loved ones. So assemble your ingredients, heat that one reliable pot or skillet, and watch how your dinner routine is transformed by the power of one-pot marvels. savor each bite!

Your culinary journey into the world of ease and flavor begins with these one-pot miracles. They are here to encourage your creativity, excite you, and serve as a reminder that a delicious dinner can be both quick to prepare and deeply fulfilling.

I appreciate you coming along with me on this journey through the world of one-pot cooking. May the smell of excellent dinners waft from your kitchen and the tyranny of dirty dishes be banished from your evenings. Here's to the miracles of one-pot wonders, which will make your life easier and your meals more enjoyable. Have fun cooking!

Chapter 6

Enhancing Your Meals with Healthy Sides

The unsung heroes of the culinary world are the side dishes. They could be in the background on your plate, but their influence on the nutritional and culinary quality of a meal cannot be understated. We'll go deeply into the world of these culinary complements in our examination of healthy sides, providing a variety of side dish dishes that feature colorful veggies, sturdy grains, and protein-rich legumes. We won't stop there, though; these sides have been designed to go well with the Chapter 4 main courses, resulting in a harmonic symphony of flavors that will have your taste buds humming.

The Importance of Side Dishes

Let's first talk about why side dishes are important parts of a balanced meal before getting into the enticing recipes.

1. Nutrient enrichment

They are nutritious powerhouses and side dishes. They offer a chance to add various vitamins, minerals, and crucial elements to your food. They can improve the overall nutritional value of your meal experience when appropriately prepared.

2.Flavor Balancing Act, second edition

In addition to nutrients, side dishes should also have flavor. They may provide contrasting textures, colors, and flavors to the main course's flavors in order to create a pleasing harmony. A tasty side dish can improve the entire dinner.

3. Diversity in Eating Habits

Dietary diversity is made possible by side dishes. They let you experiment with a variety of ingredients, such as grains, legumes, and leafy greens as well as root vegetables. This variety guarantees that you're getting a wide variety of nutrients while also keeping your palate interested.

Let's now set out on a culinary adventure through some wholesome sides that will make your meals more complete and delectable.

Colorful Vegetable Sides

When it comes to creating wholesome side dishes, vegetables are the major players. They add texture, color, and a vitamin boost to your meal. Here are some vegetable side dishes that go well with the Chapter 4 main courses:

Asparagus with Roasted Garlic and Herbs

Ingredients

Fresh asparagus spears, olive oil, and chopped garlic cloves

- Chopped fresh herbs, such as parsley, rosemary, or thyme

-Salt & pepper to taste

- Lemon zest

Instructions

1. Set the oven's temperature to 400°F (200°C).

On a baking sheet, arrange the asparagus spears.

3. Drizzle with olive oil, then top with lemon zest, fresh herbs, and chopped garlic.

4. Add salt and pepper to taste.

5. Stir to evenly coat the asparagus.

6. Roast for 10 to 12 minutes, or until fork-tender and just barely crunchy.

7. Present hot.

Relationship Suggestion: Grilled chicken or fish meals from Chapter 4 go incredibly well with the Roasted Garlic and Herb Asparagus, producing a vivid and savory combo.

Cinnamon-flavored sweet potatoes mashed

Ingredients

- Cubed, peeled, and flavored sweet potatoes

- Butter or healthy olive oil

- Cinnamon powder

- To taste, salt and pepper

Instructions

1. To make sweet potato cubes soft, steam or boil them.

194

In a bowl, mash them after draining.

3. To add richness, add a pat of butter or a drizzle of olive oil.

4. Add salt, pepper, and ground cinnamon.

5. Blend thoroughly until emulsified and creamy.

6. Use as a healthful side dish.

Relationship Suggestion: With the roast turkey or pig dishes from Chapter 4 and these Mashed

Sweet Potatoes with Cinnamon, you can make a warm and festive supper.

Legumes and Grains with Heartiness

Excellent sources of fiber, protein, and complex carbs are grains and legumes. They give your meal solidity and help you feel full. Here are a few examples of sides that highlight the adaptability of grains and legumes:

196

Salad with Quinoa and Black Beans

Ingredients

- Cooked quinoa

- Rinsed and drained black beans

- Diced red bell pepper

- Finely chopped red onion

- Chopped fresh cilantro

- Lime juice

- Cumin - Olive oil

- To taste, salt and pepper

Instructions

1. Toss cooked quinoa, black beans, diced red bell pepper, and finely sliced red onion in a large bowl.

2. To make the dressing, combine the lime juice, cumin, olive oil, salt, and pepper in a separate small bowl.

3. Smother the quinoa mixture with the dressing.

4. Add the fresh cilantro and mix everything thoroughly.

5. Present cold.

Relationship Suggestion:

Quinoa and Black Bean Salad provide a filling and protein-rich dinner when served with the grilled shrimp or tofu dishes from Chapter 4.

With cranberries and pecans, wild rice pilaf

Ingredients

- Chopped pecans, dried cranberries, and wild rice
- Minced shallots

Olive oil, fresh thyme leaves, vegetable or chicken broth, salt, and pepper to taste

Instructions

1. In a skillet, cook shallots, which have been minced, in olive oil until they are transparent.
2. Add the wild rice and keep sautéing for a few minutes.
3. Add fresh thyme leaves, vegetable or chicken broth, and salt and pepper to taste.

4. Simmer the rice with the lid on until it is cooked and has absorbed the liquid.

5. Add the chopped pecans and dried cranberries.

6. Use a fork to fluff, then serve.

Relationship Suggestion: Grilled fish or chicken meals from Chapter 4 match wonderfully with the wild rice pilaf with cranberries and pecans, providing a healthy and filling combo.

Building Harmony on Your Plate

It's time to think about how these nutritious sides can work in harmony with the main meals from Chapter 4 now that we've examined a variety of vivid vegetable sides, sturdy grains, and legumes.

Textures & Flavors in Balance

To create a harmonious dinner, flavors and textures must be balanced. Consider the contrast between a tender, flavorful main dish, and a colorful, slightly crisp vegetable side dish. Your taste senses will be treated to a pleasant experience when the flavors and textures interact.

Consider serving the Roasted Garlic and Herb Asparagus alongside, for instance, a flavorful and rich beef stir-fry from Chapter 4. The dish will be well-balanced and tasty thanks to the sharpness of the asparagus and the savory herbs.

Combinations of Colorful and Nutrient-Rich Foods

Aim for a colorful and nutrient-rich combination when selecting side dishes to serve with your main courses. A platter with a rainbow of colors often represents a wide variety of nutrition.

Serve the Quinoa and Black Bean Salad with the colorful and zesty lemon herb salmon from Chapter 4. The lime dressing in the salad will complement the salmon's zesty undertones, and the inclusion of quinoa and black beans in the dish will keep you full of protein and fiber.

Finalizing the Meal

Healthy side dishes are essential for rounding out your dinner. They complete the meal, ensuring that you are not only eating the main course but also a well-balanced plate.

Consider presenting a tasty and filling skillet dish from Chapter 4, such as a stir-fry with chicken and vegetables. Consider serving the Mashed Sweet Potatoes with

Cinnamon as a side dish to round off the dinner. The dinner feels heartier and has more depth thanks to the potatoes' creamy sweetness.

Creativity and Versatility

Healthy sides have the adaptability and possibility for creativity, which is one of their benefits. You can combine several main courses with different side dishes to make fresh flavor combinations and keep your dinners interesting.

For instance, don't be afraid to serve your favorite side dishes, such as the Wild Rice Pilaf with Cranberries and Pecans, with several main meals from Chapter 4. Its versatility can be seen in the way it can taste great with everything from grilled prawns to roast turkey.

The unsung heroes of your meals are the nutritious side dishes since they improve not just the nutritional value but also the overall eating experience. These sides have the ability to take your dish to new gastronomic heights, whether you're eating colorful vegetables, nutritious grains, or protein-rich legumes.

You'll learn the skill of creating harmony on your plate as you experiment with various pairings and combinations. It's about savoring each bite, appreciating the satisfaction of a well-balanced meal, and experiencing the variety of flavors and textures.

So gather your ingredients, check out these recipes for wholesome sides, and let your culinary imagination go wild. Healthy sides are available to make your meals complete, nourishing, and totally delicious, whether you're cooking for a weeknight dinner or hosting a large event.

There is a gourmet adventure waiting to be discovered in the world of healthy side dishes. It's a trip bursting with vivid hues, strong flavors, and the excitement of trying new pairings. We appreciate your participation as we explore the benefits of adding wholesome sides to your meals. May your dinner table be set with plates that are pleasing to the eye as well as the palate, and may your kitchen be a place of culinary inventiveness. Enjoy your adventure through food!

Chapter 7

Desserts Without Guilt: Indulging in Sweet Treats

Desserts hold a special place in both our culinary heritage and our hearts. Even the mere suggestion of sweet sweets can send our taste buds into a trance. What if, however, we told you that you can have dessert guilt-free? It's true what you just read! We're going to change the way you think about desserts in this investigation of sweets. We'll include recipes for straightforward, healthy sweets, including fruit-based options, low-sugar treats, and indulgent treats that can be enjoyed in moderation. Prepare to set out on a trip of delicious fulfillment without any remorse.

The idea behind guilt-free desserts

Before we get started with the delicious dishes, let's talk about what it means to enjoy desserts guilt-free.

1. Nourishment and Indulgence

Desserts without guilt are all about enjoying the pleasure of sweet indulgence while making decisions that support your health and Well-being objectives. It's about mindfully nurturing your body and soul, not depriving yourself.

2. Making Wise Ingredient Decisions

Smart ingredient selections are prioritized in these sweets. Healthy components including fruits, whole grains, and natural sweeteners are frequently included. You can satisfy your sweet desires without compromising your health by using these replacements.

3. Portion management

In order to enjoy guilt-free desserts, portion control is essential. You can enjoy a small slice of cake that will satisfy you without filling you up rather than devouring a huge piece. Quantity is less significant than quality.

Let's now tempt your taste buds with some sweet treat dishes that personify pleasure without feeling bad.

Fresh Fruit Delights

Fruits are the basis for many guilt-free treats and are nature's lovely gift to us. Along with a variety of vitamins, fiber, and antioxidants, they offer natural sugars. Here are a few sweets made of fruit that will sate your hunger guilt-free:

Apples with cinnamon and walnuts baked in the oven

Ingredients

- Apples (choose your preferred variety)
- Cinnamon, ground
- Walnuts, chopped
- Optional sprinkle of honey or maple syrup
- Optional nutmeg sprinkling

Instructions

1. Set the oven's temperature to 375°F (190°C).

2. Keep the apple bottoms on while coring the fruit.

In a baking dish, put the apples.

4. Top each apple with ground cinnamon and chopped walnuts.

5. If you would like more sweetness, drizzle with honey or maple syrup.

6. Add a small amount of nutmeg for flavor.

7. Bake the apples in the oven for about 25 to 30 minutes, or until they are soft.

8. Present warm, and savor.

Relationship Suggestion: Warm Baked Apples go perfectly with a dab of Greek yogurt or a scoop of vanilla frozen yogurt, creating a lovely contrast of temps and textures.

Greek yogurt parfait with berries

Ingredients

- Strawberries, blueberries, and raspberries mixed together

- Greek yogurt, either plain or flavored to your taste

- Granola (choose a version with less sugar)

- Fresh mint leaves (to use as a garnish)

Instructions

1. Arrange Greek yogurt, mixed berries, and granola in a glass or bowl.

2. Continue layering until the bowl or glass is full.

3. Add a dollop of yogurt and a garnish of fresh mint to complete the dish.

4. Present cold.

Consider these pairings: Your Berry Parfait can be enhanced with a drizzle of honey or a garnish of dark chocolate shavings for an additional sweet and sophisticated touch.

Sugar-Free Temptations

Sugar reduction does not equate to flavor reduction. Desserts made with less sugar show that it's possible to experience sweetness in its purest form. Here are a few delights that have perfected the low-sugar indulgence technique:

Avocado Dark Chocolate Mousse

Ingredients

-Ripe avocados and bitter chocolate powder

- A dash of almond milk - A drizzle of honey or maple syrup

A dash of salt and vanilla extract

Instructions

Smooth and creamy results can be achieved by blending ripe avocados with dark chocolate powder, honey or maple syrup, almond milk, vanilla extract, and a dash of salt.

2. Add extra honey or cocoa to your preferred level of sweetness and chocolate intensity.

3. Put the mousse in the fridge for at least an hour to chill.

4. Dish out little servings.

Relationship Suggestion:

Toppings for your Dark Chocolate Avocado Mousse can include whipped cream or a sprinkling of chopped pistachios.

Cookies with chocolate chips and oats

Ingredients

- Whole wheat flour - Dark chocolate chips - Rolled oats (Select a variety that has at least 70% cocoa)

- Applesauce without sugar

- Olive oil or coconut oil

- A tiny bit of honey or maple syrup

- 1/8 teaspoon of cinnamon

- Baked soda

- A dash of salt

Instructions

1. In a bowl, combine whole wheat flour, rolled oats, dark chocolate chips, applesauce that hasn't been sweetened, coconut oil or olive oil, honey or maple syrup, a dash of cinnamon, baking soda, and salt.

2. Scoop out little balls of cookie dough and press them onto a baking sheet.

3. Bake for 10 to 12 minutes, or until golden brown, in an oven that has been prepared to 350°F (175°C).

4. Permit to cool, then moderately consume.

Relationship Suggestion: The cozy aromas of these oatmeal chocolate chip cookies can be complemented with a glass of chilled almond milk or a cup of herbal tea.

Indulgences with Portion Control

A secret weapon for sweets that are guilt-free is portion management. These sweets are created to quench your desire for sweetness without overpowering your senses. Here are a few delightful possibilities:

Cheesecake bites in miniature

Ingredients

- Low-fat cream cheese.

- Plain or flavoring Greek yogurt

A tiny bit of honey or maple syrup

- Crumbled Graham Crackers

- Fresh berries (as a garnish)

Instructions

1. In a mixing bowl, combine Greek yogurt, honey, or maple syrup, reduced-fat cream cheese, and stir until well combined.

2. Use paper liners to line a muffin pan.

3. Fill the base of each liner with Graham Cracker crumbs.

4. Spread the graham cracker layer with the cream cheese mixture.

5. Allow it to chill for at least an hour in the fridge.

6. Before serving, top each small cheesecake with fresh berries.

Relationship Suggestion: Your Mini Cheesecake Bites can be made a little more decadent by adding a drizzle of chocolate sauce or a garnish of crushed nuts.

Strawberry-Covered in Chocolate

Ingredients

- Strawberry freshness
- Dark chocolate (choose a type with at least 70% cocoa content).
- Optional chopped nuts for coating

Instructions

1. Use a double boiler or a microwave to melt the dark chocolate.

2. Coat fresh strawberries half or completely with melted chocolate.

3. Arrange the chocolate-covered strawberries on a dish covered with parchment paper.

4. If preferred, top with chopped nuts.

5. Chill the strawberries for around 30 minutes to help the chocolate solidify.

6. Present and savor.

Relationship Suggestion: The taste of chocolate-covered

strawberries can be enhanced by a glass of sparkling water or a crisp, fruity white wine.

Desserts are meant to be a pleasurable part of life's culinary journey, not a guilty pleasure. You may indulge in the romance of desserts without sacrificing your health with the help of these recipes for guilt-free sweet treats. There is a sweet treat for every occasion, whether you choose fruit-based treats, low-sugar temptations, or portion-controlled indulgences.

As you examine these recipes, keep in mind that moderation and thoughtful decisions are the keys to enjoyment that is guilt-free. Enjoy the delights in every bite and the satisfaction of dessert without feeling guilty.

The options are boundless in the world of sweet delicacies, where tastes and imagination are unrestricted. We appreciate you joining us as we explore desserts without guilt. May you enjoy the taste of ripe fruits, the scent of freshly baked cookies, and the pleasure of sharing sweets with loved ones. Enjoy your guilt-free foray into the realm of desserts!

Chapter 8

Revitalize Your Sip: Quick and Nutritious Drinks

The key to good health is being hydrated, and the beverages we select can have a big impact. Welcome to the world of fast, nourishing drinks. Here, we'll discuss the value of staying hydrated and enjoying the pleasure of sipping a variety of hydrating, nutritional drinks. We'll go through smoothies, fresh juice, herbal tea, and infused water recipes on this voyage, all of which are meant to keep you hydrated and fed from the inside out.

The Importance of Drinking Plenty of Water

Before we explore the lovely world of healthy beverages, let's take a moment to comprehend why maintaining hydration is so important.

1. Essential for Survival

For our bodies to work correctly, hydration is crucial. Water is necessary for the function of every cell, tissue, and organ. The biological machinery in our bodies depends on it to function properly.

2. Vigor and Concentration

Fatigue and impaired cognitive function are two effects of dehydration. You can maintain your energy levels and mental clarity throughout the day by drinking enough water.

3. Facilitating Digestion

By ensuring that our digestive organs operate at their best, enough hydration helps digestion.

It aids in digestion, nutrient absorption, and waste removal.

4. Glowing Skin

Skin that is healthy and radiant can benefit from proper hydration. It promotes a young complexion, lowers the danger of dryness, and maintains skin elasticity.

5. Detoxification

A natural detoxifier is water. It supports general detoxification and a strong immune system by aiding in the removal of waste products and toxins from the body.

After learning how crucial it is to stay hydrated, let's look at some drinks that can not only quench your thirst but also provide several health advantages.

Smoothies with a lot of nutrients

Smoothies are a great way to blend different ingredients to create a tasty and nutrient-rich beverage. They are adaptable options at any time of day because they provide limitless customization options.

Smoothie with green goddess

Ingredients

- Leaves from spinach or kale

- Banana

- Plain or flavoring Greek yogurt

- Almond milk (or the milk of your choice).

the Chia seed

- Optional honey for extra sweetness

Instructions

1. Blend spinach or kale leaves, a ripe banana, Greek yogurt, almond milk, chia seeds, and any more honey you like in a blender.

2. Blend until creamy and smooth.

3. Pour into a glass, then take a sip.

Health Advantages: This Green Goddess Smoothie is a nutritious powerhouse. Vitamins and antioxidants are found in spinach or kale, while potassium and natural sweetness are found in bananas. Chia seeds give you fiber and omega-3 fatty acids, while Greek yogurt gives you probiotics and protein.

Fresh Juices Packed With Fruit

A lively and revitalizing way to experience the goodness of fruits and vegetables is through freshly squeezed juices. They are a great complement to your daily routine because they offer a rich dose of vitamins and minerals.

Citrus Juice Sunrise
Ingredients
- Carrots
- Oranges

- Ginger, if desired

- A tiny bit of honey, if desired

Instructions:

1. Peel and cut carrots and oranges into bite-sized pieces.

2. For a zingy kick, if preferred, add a tiny slice of ginger.

3. Use a juicer to extract the ingredients.

4. If necessary, add a little honey to sweeten.

5. Pour into a glass, then take a sip to appreciate the dawn.

Health Advantages: Oranges, which are a great source of vitamin C, are combined with beta-carotene and fiber from carrots in the Sunrise Citrus Juice. Honey provides natural sweetness, while ginger adds a natural spice and has digestive benefits.

Relaxing herbal teas

In addition to being calming, herbal teas offer several health advantages. Herbal teas can help you when you want a soothing cup before bed or a reviving sip in the morning.

Tea with chamomile and lavender
Ingredients
- Loose or bagged chamomile tea

- Fresh or dried lavender buds - Hot water

Instructions

1. As directed on the packaging, steep a chamomile tea bag or loose tea in boiling water.

2. Sprinkle a few lavender buds into the tea as it steeps.

3. Permit an additional two to three minutes for the tea to brew.

4. Discard the tea bag or brew the loose tea.

5. Take a sip and allow the calming aroma to calm your senses.

Health Advantages Because of its well-known relaxing effects, chamomile tea is a great option for unwinding and falling asleep. The addition of lavender gives the tea a peaceful and aromatic depth that intensifies its sedative properties.

Rejuvenating Infused Water

A revitalizing method to step up your hydration is with infused water. You may improve the flavor of water and gain additional health advantages by infusing it with fruits, herbs, and spices.

Water With Mint and Cucumber Ingredients

- Cucumber slices
- Fresh mint
- Cold water

- Cubes of ice

Instructions

1. Fill a pitcher with fresh mint leaves and cucumber slices.
2. Fill the pitcher with ice cubes and cold water.
3. Gently stir the ingredients and allow them to steep for at least an hour.
4. Pour into glasses, then inhale the crisp, cooling flavor of the cucumber and mint.

Health Advantages: Water with cucumber and mint is hydrating as well as refreshing. Cucumbers contain a lot of water, and mint adds a flavorful burst and may help with digestion.

Establishing a Hydration Schedule

After learning about these convenient and nourishing beverages, it's critical to develop a hydration habit that works for you.

Here are some pointers to keep you on course:

1. Establish daily objectives:
Set a goal to consume a certain amount of water every day. Depending on your needs and degree of activity, this could be 8 glasses (64 ounces) or more.

2.Always keep a reusable bottle on you: Always have a reusable water bottle with you. It helps as a prompt to frequently consume water.

3. Flavorful Selection: To keep hydration fun, try out various healthy beverages. Alternate between herbal teas, smoothies, fresh juices, and infused water.

4. Schedule Hydration: To maintain consistency, set phone reminders or use applications that monitor your water intake.

5. Listen to Your Body: Pay attention to the cues coming from your body. It's important to hydrate when you're thirsty.

Drinking healthy beverages and staying hydrated can significantly improve your well-being. In addition to quenching your thirst, these beverages provide your body with vital nutrients and antioxidants. Every beverage has its special advantages, whether you're starting your day with a

Green Goddess Smoothie, reviving with a Sunrise Citrus Juice, unwinding with a Chamomile Lavender Tea, or sipping on Cucumber and Mint Infused Water.

Remember that it's not just about water; it's about self-care and nourishment as you enjoy the world of fast and healthy drinks. These beverages are a tasty and fun approach to providing your body with the greatest care possible.

The voyage of fast-acting, wholesome drinks is delightful. Each drink is an opportunity to rejuvenate your body and soul on this exploration voyage. We appreciate your participation as we investigate hydration and tasty nourishment. May the refreshing coolness of cucumber and mint, the energizing vitality of Sunrise Citrus Juice, and the calming serenity of Chamomile Lavender Tea fill your days. Have fun exploring the world of fast and wholesome drinks!

Chapter 9

Planning and preparing meals with ease

Meal planning and preparation are often neglected in the flurry of modern living. Nevertheless, they are crucial resources for sustaining a healthy and balanced diet. Welcome to the world of meal planning and preparation. We'll help you create a meal plan that fits your lifestyle, give you an example menu plan using recipes from earlier chapters, and offer advice on how to shop and prepare meals quickly. By the time this adventure is over, you'll be equipped with the information and abilities needed to prepare meals on your own, save time, and make healthier decisions.

The Science of Meal Preparation

Meal planning functions as a kind of gastronomic voyage map. It enables you to plan your meals, decrease food waste, and make wise dietary decisions. Meal planning can be customized to meet your specific lifestyle, whether you're a busy professional, student, or parent.

1. Examine your schedule

Examine your weekly calendar to start. Do you prefer to cook on days when you have more time or on nights when you need quick fixes? You may plan meals that are useful for your life by having a clear understanding of your timetable.

2. Identify Your Goals

Take into account your dietary habits and goals. Do you want to maintain your weight, follow a balanced diet, or meet certain nutritional needs? Do you have any dietary preferences or limits, such as being a vegetarian or avoiding gluten? Your food plan will be influenced by your interests and goals.

3. Select Your Recipes

Choose recipes now that fit your schedule, objectives, and preferences. You can use the recipes we've discussed in earlier chapters, such as the Stir-Fried Chicken and Vegetables for a filling dinner or the Green Goddess Smoothie for a quick breakfast.

4. Make a weekly schedule.

Make a weekly food plan using your recipes as a guide. Put a specific day and mealtime for each recipe. Be adaptable and think about using leftovers or meals that can be used another day.

5. Create a grocery list

Make a list of the ingredients you'll need for your shopping trip based on your meal plan. To make your grocery shopping easier, group the list by category (such as produce, dairy products, and pantry essentials).

Sample Weekly Meal Schedule

Let's use a sample weekly meal plan to put the meal planning procedure into practice. This menu includes dishes from earlier chapters to show how to put

together a well-rounded and
balanced diet.

Day 1: Monday.

Green Goddess Smoothie for
breakfast (Chapter 6)
Quinoa and black bean salad for
lunch (Chapter 4)
(Chapter 4) "Dinner: Baked
Salmon with Lemon Herb Sauce"
Fruit, fresh fruit

Day 2: Tuesday

Overnight oats with berries for breakfast (Chapter 4)

Wild rice pilaf with cranberries and pecans (Chapter 4) is served for lunch.

Dinner will be a stir-fried chicken dish with broccoli and cashews (Chapter 4).

Greek yogurt and honey as a snack

Day 3: Wednesday.

Oatmeal chocolate chip cookies
for breakfast (Chapter 7)
Lunch: Asparagus with Roasted
Garlic and Herbs (Chapter 4)
One-pot spaghetti with Tomato
Sauce for dinner (Chapter 5)
Cucumber slices with hummus as
a snack

Day 4: Thursday.

Berry Parfait with Greek Yogurt for
Breakfast (Chapter 6)
(Chapter 4) "Lunch:" Mashed
Sweet Potatoes with Cinnamon
Dinner: Sheet pan dinner of beef
and vegetables (Chapter 5)
Mixed nuts as a snack

Day 5: Friday.

Breakfast: Strawberries with a
chocolate coating (Chapter 7)

Spinach and Mixed Berry Salad for lunch (Chapter 4)

One-pot chickpea and Vegetable Curry for dinner (Chapter 5)

Fruit, fresh fruit

Day 6: Saturday.

Scrambled eggs with spinach and feta for breakfast; leftover chickpea and vegetable curry for lunch; grilled shrimp over quinoa for dinner (Chapter 4).

Hummus and sliced bell peppers for a snack

Sunday: Day 7.

Breakfast: Fruit Salad with Honey-Lime Dressing (Chapter 4) Lunch: One-pot spaghetti with Tomato Sauce that was made in advance (Chapter 4)
Dinner: Baked Chicken with a Herb Crust (Chapter 4)
Greek yogurt with berries as a snack

Shopping for groceries effectively

Effective meal planning and preparation start with efficient grocery shopping. Here are some pointers to help you maximize your grocery store visits:

Adhere to Your List

Review your menu and shopping list before you leave for the store.

276

You may avoid impulsive purchases and stay within your spending limit by following your list.

Visit the Perimeter

Fresh produce, dairy products, and proteins are typically found around the outside of grocery stores. Pay attention to these places because they frequently have whole, unprocessed foods.

Purchase in bulk

Consider purchasing in bulk for pantry essentials like rice, pasta, and canned foods. This can help you save money over time and make fewer trips to the store.

Opt for seasonal produce

Where feasible, choose seasonal fruits and vegetables. They frequently have more flavor, are cheaper, and are fresher.

Additionally, they provide your meals with diversity.

Price Comparison

Compare pricing and think about store brands or generic alternatives. You might discover that they provide comparable quality for less money.

Eat less processed food

Reduce the amount of packaged and processed foods you buy. These foods typically have more added sugars, salt, and bad fats. Place an emphasis on natural, complete ingredients.

Prepare for leftovers

Make sure to incorporate repurposed leftovers in your meal plans. For instance, if you roast a chicken, the leftovers can be used in stir-fries, salads, or sandwiches.

The Influence of Meal Planning

The last step in ensuring that your meal planning efforts result in simple, healthy meals is meal preparation. You may save time on hectic weekdays and make eating healthy simple by setting aside some time for meal preparation.

1. Select Your Prep Day

Choose a day during the week when you have a little extra time to spend on meal preparation. This might happen on a Sunday afternoon or any other day that works for you.

2. Collect Your Tools

Make sure you have the right kitchenware for meal preparation, such as cutting boards, mixing bowls, storage containers, and kitchen appliances like a food processor or blender.

3. Clean and Chop

Peeling, washing, and slicing produce should come first. During the week, you may use these for salads, snacks, or quick stir-fries.

4. Cook in Groups

Prepare large quantities of pasta or grains like quinoa. Prepare proteins like meat, chicken, or beans ahead of time. You'll have the ingredients for a variety of dinners if you do it this way.

5. Portion and Store

Make portion-sized containers out of your prepared components. On busy days, it is simple to grab and put together meals as a result. To preserve freshness, date-mark containers.

6. Preparation of Snacks

Prepare wholesome snacks like yogurt cups, cut-up fruit, or pre-portioned nuts. Having these snacks on hand can help you avoid reaching for less healthy options.

Accept Freezer Meals, number seven

Prepare dishes that can be frozen in advance. You may portion out and freeze soups, stews, and casseroles for later use.

Combining Everything

It's time to put what you've learned about the art of meal planning and preparation into practice. Make your food plan first, taking into account your interests, goals, and lifestyle. Take ideas from the suggested weekly meal plan, and don't be afraid to get inventive with your cooking.

You'll find that making healthful meals is easier to manage and takes less time when you buy wisely and meal plan like a master. This method of meal planning and preparation will eventually turn into a useful habit that benefits your health and well-being.

Keep in mind that meal preparation is a versatile tool. You are welcome to modify it as your schedule and preferences change. Making healthy eating a sustainable and joyful aspect of your life is the aim.

Not only can meal preparation and planning help you feed your body, but they also help you nourish your spirit and make your daily routine simpler. They provide you the power to make wise dietary decisions, save time in the kitchen, and ultimately live a better and more well-rounded life.

I hope that this exploration of the world of meal preparation and planning has given you the information and motivation to start your culinary journey. Whether you're cooking for a family dinner, a special event, or a workday lunch, may your kitchen be a place of inspiration and nourishment? Enjoy the advantages of thoughtful meal preparation and savor each delectable bite.

Conclusion
Embracing Simpleness: A Satisfying Ending

It's time to relish the pleasures of our shared culinary excursion and consider how straightforward cooking with fewer ingredients is as we come to the end of our culinary voyage through "Skinnytaste Simple Cookbook: Quick and Wholesome Dishes with Minimal Ingredients." We've discovered a world of delicious recipes in these pages that demonstrate you don't need a lengthy list of ingredients to make a filling and healthy supper. As we continue on this delectable journey, let's review our main lessons, encourage you to adopt a healthier and more practical eating style, and ask for your insightful comments.

Key Takeaways: Simplicity Is Everything

We've come across a wealth of knowledge along the way that highlights the beauty of simplicity in cooking:

Quality Over Quantity

With fewer components, the quality of each component is more heavily emphasized. By using healthful, fresh ingredients, you can enhance the flavors of your food without adding needless complications.

Time-Saving Magic

Saving time in the kitchen is another aspect of cooking with simplicity that goes beyond the ingredients. We've shown you how to make wonderful meals with our recipes without spending all day at the stove.

Flexible Creations

You may make a variety of foods that fit your diet and lifestyle with just a few simple components. Our cookbook has demonstrated that simplicity has no limitations, from breakfast to dessert.

Mindful Consumption

Adopting simplicity promotes attentiveness when eating. You get a deeper appreciation for the flavors and nourishment each dish offers by relishing the dishes' fewer ingredients.

Adopt a Healthier and More Convenient Eating Habit

More than just a cookbook, "Skinnytaste Simple" is a journey that invites you to change the way you eat and view food. Here are some tips for adopting a more practical and healthy eating style:

1. Organize Your Pantry

Examine your refrigerator and pantry in more detail. Exist products with extensive ingredient lists or synthetic additives? Think about switching them out for full, unprocessed options.

2. Plan strategically

Meal planning is your secret weapon for eating healthy, as we've covered in a separate chapter. Make meal plans that are in line with your objectives, then use them to direct your grocery and meal preparation.

3. Mindful Servings

Eat meals that are portion-controlled. You can indulge in your favorite meals while still eating a balanced diet if you are aware of your portion proportions.

4. Drink Water Mindfully

Keep hydrated with quick and filling beverages like those we've listed. A crucial component of well-being that is frequently ignored is hydration.

5. Try New Things and Adapt

Don't be hesitant to play around with the recipes you've learned here. Explore new ingredients, give dishes your spin, and tweak recipes to your liking. You are the artist; cooking is an art.

Invite Comments and Further Research

The last page of this cookbook doesn't mark the conclusion of our culinary journey. Your comments will be extremely helpful in determining future editions and products. We encourage you to contribute your opinions, stories, and any ideas you may have.

Resources for Additional Research

Take a look at these resources as you continue your culinary exploration and delve into the world of healthy and straightforward cooking:

1. Cooking Workshops and Classes

Look into any nearby cooking classes or workshops. Your culinary abilities can be improved, and you'll learn new cooking methods thanks to these practical encounters.

2. Communities that Cook

Connect with other foodies by joining online cooking

communities and forums. It can be entertaining and educational to learn from others and share experiences.

3. Investigate Cookbooks

There are a plethora of cookbooks available, each presenting its own perspective on the culinary arts. Look into other cookbooks that share your passion for cooking.

As we say goodbye to our culinary journey, keep in mind that cooking simply is a way to nourish, harmony, and joy. Accept it wholeheartedly and allow it to lead you on a path to more flavorful, convenient, and healthy eating. These recipes are just the start of your culinary journey, and we can't wait to follow you on your culinary excursions.

I appreciate you coming along on this wonderful journey with

"Skinnytaste Simple Cookbook." You've only just started on your path to a tastier and healthier diet. May you have easy-to-make meals with fresh ingredients, and may the perfume of healthful goodness fill your house.

Happy cooking and bon appetit until we cross paths again in the world of culinary adventure!

Appendices
Your Culinary Reference
Guide

Your best ally in the realm of cooking is information. Having access to useful information may make a world of difference, whether you're a seasoned chef or just starting on your culinary path. A reference cookbook that will be your go-to in the kitchen is presented in this section.

Consider this your culinary toolset, complete with a dictionary of terms for basic cooking as well as conversion tables and measurement equivalents for our international readers.

Beginner's Glossary of Cooking Terms

Cooking has its vocabulary, which contains words and expressions that newcomers may find difficult to understand. Don't worry; we're here to assist you in understanding the vocabulary of the kitchen. To help you in your culinary explorations, the following vocabulary of terms related to cooking is provided:

1. Bake: To bake meals in a dry, enclosed environment. For bread, cakes, and casseroles, this technique is frequently applied.

2. To boil is to heat a liquid to the degree at which it begins to bubble ferociously. commonly applied to veggies, potatoes, and pasta.

3. Sauté: To swiftly cook food over high heat in a tiny amount of oil or butter. For vegetables and meat, this technique is frequently employed.

4. Simmer: To gently prepare food by simmering it in liquid until just barely boiling. For sauces, stews, and soups, this technique works well.

5. Grill: To cook food on a grill or over an open flame. Foods like steak, chicken, and vegetables have a smokey flavor and appealing grill marks when they are grilled.

6. Roast: To use dry heat to cook food in an oven, usually with the door open. For vegetables, poultry, and meats, this technique works well.

7. Blanch: To stop cooking food by temporarily submerging it in boiling water and then moving it right away to ice-cold water. frequently applied to vegetables.

8. Sear: To quickly sear the meat over high heat to brown the surface. Cooking over heat keeps liquids in and improves flavor.

9. Dice: To create uniformly sized, tiny food cubes.

10 Julienne: To thinly slice food into strips similar to matchsticks.

11. Mince: To very precisely slice food into very little pieces.

12. Grate; To use a grater to grind food into tiny pieces. used frequently with cheese and veggies.

13. The zest is the bitter, outer layer of citrus fruit peel. It is used to give foods a burst of citrus taste.

14. Whip: Beat things vigorously to incorporate air and produce a light, fluffy texture, typically eggs or cream.

15. Fold: To gently stir two ingredients together, usually by lifting and twisting a spatula. To maintain a delicate, airy texture, this is done.

16. Deglazing is the process of adding liquid to a pan of food that has been roasted or sautéed to remove the tasty browned bits that have clung to the bottom.

17. Reduce: Heat a beverage to a simmer so that the flavor is enhanced and the consistency is thickened.

18. Baste: To add flavor and moisture to food by spooning juices or liquid over it while it cooks.

19. Blanch: To quickly cease cooking food by immersing it in icy water after briefly cooking it in boiling water.

20. Dredge: before cooking, dust food—usually meat or fish—with a dry substance like flour or breadcrumbs.

This glossary provides a good place to start when learning common culinary terms. You'll come across additional terminology as you go deeper into the realm of food, adding to your culinary vocabulary.

Conversion tables and measurement equivalents are provided.

Precision measurements are essential for producing consistent and delicious outcomes because cooking is both an art and a science. However, there are numerous measurement methods in use around the globe, making it challenging to follow recipes from various sources. We've put up-conversion tables and measurement equivalents to make navigating the world of cooking easier and to make your culinary adventure more enjoyable.

Volume measurements include:

- One tablespoon equals three tablespoons
- Two teaspoons equal one fluid ounce (fl oz).
- 1 cup = 8 ounces of liquid
- 2 cups equal 1 pint (pt).

- 4 cups make up 1 quart (qt).

- 4 quarts make up 1 gallon (gal)

Dry measurements are:

1 ounce (oz) is equal to 28.35 grams (g).

- 16 ounces make up one pound (lb).

- A kilo (kg) is equal to 2.205 pounds.

Temperature conversions

include:

- Converting from Fahrenheit to Celsius: (°F - 32) 5/9 = °C
- Converting from Celsius to Fahrenheit: (C 9/5) + 32 = °F

Examples of Common Ingredient Equivalents

- 1 stick of butter is equivalent to 1/2 cup, 8 tablespoons, and 4 ounces.
- 120 grams are in 1 cup of all-purpose flour.
- 200 grams in 1 cup of granulated sugar
- 220 grams in 1 cup of brown sugar

240 milliliters (ml) make up one cup of milk.

240 ml make up 1 cup of vegetable oil.

- 180 grams are in 1 cup of rice.

- 90 grams in 1 cup of oats

Temperature conversions for ovens

350°F is equivalent to 180°C, 375°F to 190°C, 400°F to 200°C, 425°F to 220°C, and 450°F to 230°C.

Conversions from Imperial to Metric

- 1 liter (L) = 33.8 fluid ounces = 4 cups
- 1 milliliter (ml) = 0.034 fluid ounces
- 100 ml = 3.38 fluid ounces
- 250 ml = 8.45 fluid ounces
- 500 ml = 16.9 fluid ounces

Conversions from cups to grams (common ingredients)

- Flour: One cup equals 120 grams
- Granulated sugar: 1 cup equals 200 grams
- Brown sugar: 1 cup equals 220 grams

Ounce to Gram Conversions:

- 25 grams are equivalent to 0.88 ounces, 50 grams to 1.76 ounces,

100 grams to 3.53 ounces, 250 grams to 8.82 ounces to equal half a pound, and 500 grams to equal one pound.